Achieving realistic fitness goals: A guide to Sustainable fitness goals for beginners.

Callie M. Henley

ABOUT THE AUTHOR

Introducing Callie M. Henley, an esteemed fitness expert committed to revolutionizing the way we approach health and wellness. With a profound interest in sustainable fitness goals, she stands at the forefront of a movement that values long-term well-being over quick fixes.

With a wealth of experience in the fitness industry, she has honed her skills in designing holistic and achievable fitness plans. Her approach goes beyond mere physical transformations, emphasizing the importance of balance, consistency, and environmentally conscious practices.

Guided by a passion for sustainability, she not only helps individuals reach their fitness aspirations but also promotes a lifestyle that respects the planet. Her programs incorporate eco-friendly practices, fostering a harmonious connection between personal health and environmental well-being.

In a world often dominated by short-lived trends, she champions the cause of lasting change. Her expertise empowers clients to set realistic goals, building habits that stand the test of time. Join her on a transformative journey towards a healthier, happier, and more sustainable life — where fitness is not just a goal but a sustainable lifestyle choice.

INTRODUCTION

Forget the torture of lifting heavy metals and eating fancy meals! This is not a crash course to a chiseled physique, but a blueprint for building a lasting love affair with your body. We're ditching the unrealistic pressure and embracing the slow, steady climb towards sustainable fitness goals that fit your life like a comfy pair of sneakers.

In this guide, you'll leave behind the "all-or-nothing" mentality and discover the joy of micro-victories. We'll explore the power of personalized goals, crafting ambitions that ignite your passion, not your anxiety. You'll learn to listen to your body's wisdom, building a healthy rhythm of movement and rest that nourishes your soul as much as your muscles.

Forget quick fixes and fad diets. This is about nurturing a fit lifestyle that integrates seamlessly into your daily routine. We'll delve into smart nutrition, fun workout ideas, and strategies for conquering common roadblocks. It's about finding activities you crave, not routines you dread.

So, whether your aspirations are running a marathon or simply climbing the stairs with less huff and puff, this guide is your compass. Let's embark on a fitness journey that's less about achieving a destination and more about loving the journey itself.

Get ready to ditch the guilt, celebrate the small wins, and build a fit, vibrant life that's sustainable for the long haul. Your body will thank you for it.

Chapter 1: Misconceptions about Weight Loss

• Dispelling Common Myths in Fitness

We've all heard the whispers: "carbs are evil," "skip breakfast for faster results," or "one magic smoothie does it all." But when it comes to weight loss, truth be told, most of what's buzzing around is pure myth, myth, myth!

So, let's clear the air and set the record straight. Here's a quick bust of some common weight loss misconceptions:

Myth #1: Carbs are the enemy: Nope! Carbs are our body's main fuel source. Ditching them completely can leave you feeling drained and grumpy. Choose whole grains, fruits, and veggies over processed carbs, and fuel your body right!

Myth #2: Skip meals to shrink: Uh-oh, rebound city! Skipping meals messes with your metabolism and triggers hunger pangs, leading you to overeat later. Three balanced meals and healthy snacks are the way to go.

Myth #3: Crash diets are the golden ticket: Think quick fix, think quick crash. These extreme diets are unsustainable and unhealthy. Aim for slow, steady progress with sustainable changes to your eating and exercise habits.

Myth #4: More training: Don't overdo it! Overtraining can lead to injuries and burnout. Find a balance of challenging workouts with rest days to recover and rebuild muscle.

Myth #5: Magic potions and pills do the trick: Sorry, potions are for Harry Potter, not weight loss. No shortcut can replace a healthy diet and regular exercise. Be wary of quick-fix pills and powders, they're more likely to empty your wallet than your belly.

Myth #6: Eating late equals weight gain: Time doesn't matter as much as what you eat. Focus on overall calorie intake and healthy meal choices, not the clock on the wall.

Myth #7: All calories are created equal: Not so fast! A slice of cake vs. a bowl of oatmeal have the same calorie count, but their impact on your body is different. Choose nutrient-rich foods over empty calories for sustained energy and overall health.

Remember, weight loss is a personal journey. Focus on making healthy choices that fit your lifestyle and listen to your body. Ditch the myths, embrace the facts, and enjoy the rewarding experience of building a sustainable, healthy you!

• Understanding Healthy Weight Management

Forget crash diets and quick fixes. Healthy weight operation is not a sprint, it's a marathon of smart choices and sustainable habits. Let's gutter the pressure and embrace a balanced approach that nourishes your body and energies your soul.

Here are some ways to help you understand healthy weight management :

1. Know your friend, the calorie: Understand what energies your body, but do not obsess over figures. Focus on quality over volume, choosing nutrient-rich whole foods over reused options.
2. Befriend movement, not the routine: Find activities you enjoy, from brisk walks to Zumba classes. Make it a daily ritual, not a chore and watch your energy situations soar.
3. Listen to your body's language: Ditch restrictive rules and embrace intuitive eating. Learn to recognize hunger cues and malnutrition signals, nourishing your body when it needs it, not by the timepiece.
4. Sleep tight, weight right: Rest is your body's reset button. Prioritize quality sleep for optimal hormone balance and metabolism regulation.
5. Stress less, move more: Habitual stress can sabotage your weight operations. Find healthy ways to deal with stress, from yoga to meditation, and watch your body respond appreciatively.

6. Celebrate non-scale wins: Weight loss is not just about the number on the scale. Focus on how you feel, your increased energy, and your stronger body. Every healthy choice is a win!

Remember , this is your trip, not a competition. Embrace progress, not perfection. Make small, sustainable changes and watch them balloon into a healthier, happier you. Your body will thank you for it!

Chapter 2: Psychology Behind Fitness

Fitness is not just about sculpted abs and toned biceps; it's an internal game too. Understanding the psychology behind fitness can be the key to unleashing your full potential and your relationship with movement.

Here are some ways to understand the psychology behind fitness:

1. Provocation matters: Forget crash diets and unrealistic prospects. rather, find your" why." What sparks your passion for movement? Is it feeling strong and confident? Reducing stress? Boosting energy? Connecting with nature? When you connect to a deeper purpose, exercise becomes less of a chore and further of a joyous pursuit.

2. Mind over muscle: Your studies have immense power over your body. Positive self- talk, visualization ways, and celebrating small triumphs can fuel your exercises and push you through challenges. Rather than focusing on negatives, like fatigue or mistrustfulness, shift your focus to your strengths and adaptability.

3. Embrace the inflow: Remember that feeling of being" in the zone" during a drill? That is the power of an inflow state, where you are completely immersed in the present moment, free from distractions and self- judgment. Chancing conditioning that challenges you yet feel royal can unleash this state of complete immersion and lead to deeper enjoyment.

4. Make it social: Working out with a friend, joining a group fitness class, or changing an online community can give precious support and responsibility. Social connections can boost provocation, make exercises further fun, and keep you on track towards your pretensions.

5. Reward yourself wisely: Ditch the junk food feasts. Rather, award yourself with things you truly value, like spending time in nature, taking a comforting bath, or reading a good book. Focus on prices that nourish your mind and spirit, promoting a more holistic approach to well- being.

6. Reframe your mindset: Stop seeing exercise as discipline or a chore. Rather, view it as a form of self - care, a gift you give yourself to move your body,

boost your mood, and invest in your long- term health. Shift your perspective and watch your relationship with fitness blossom.

Remember the psychology of fitness is a trip, not a destination. Discover what works for you, and celebrate every step along the way. By understanding the mind-muscle connection, you can unleash a world of possibilities of exercise from a struggle to a source of joy, commission, and lasting well- being.

● Building a Positive Mindset for Change

To develop a positive mindset, you need to shift your focus from what you" should" do to what you" want" to do. When you frame goods as scores, you set ourselves up for resistance and negativity. Rather, take time to reflect and remind yourself why this change matters to you. Is it about feeling healthier, being more confident, or achieving a particular thing? Connecting with your deeper conjurations will fuel your decisiveness and make the process more enjoyable.

Here are some ways to develop a positive mindset

1. Embrace small triumphs: Don't get discouraged by the enormity of your thing. Break it down into a lower, attainable way and celebrate each corner along the way. Completing amini- drill, cooking a healthy mess, or simply saying" no" to temptation are all triumphs worth admitting. recognizing your progress, no matter how incremental, will keep you motivated and moving forward.
2. Challenge negative thoughts : We all have an inner critic, but it doesn't have to control the narrative. When self- distrustfulness creeps in, challenge those negative studies with positive affirmations. Remind yourself of your strengths, formerly successes, and the reasons why you're embarking on this change in the first place. Positive self- talk can be an important tool for silencing negativity and boosting your confidence.
3. Find your support system: Partake your trip with buddies, family, or a supportive online community. Having friends in your corner can give a sense of responsibility, especially when challenges arise.

4. Exercise appreciativeness: Take time each day to appreciate the good goods in your life, big or small. Whether it's a mess, a beautiful evening, or simply the fact that you woke up healthy, focusing on appreciativeness can shift your mindset from lack to cornucopia. This positive outlook will unmask over into your sweats to change, making the trip feel more fulfilling.

5. Be kind to yourself: Change is a process, and there will be falls along the way. Don't beat yourself up over setbacks or occasional indulgences. rather, practice tone- compassion and see them as learning openings. Forgive yourself, get back on track, and flash reverse that progress, not perfection, is the key to lasting change.

6. Visualize success: Take numerous beats each day to close your eyes and imagine yourself achieving your thing. See yourself feeling confident, healthy, and happy. This internal exercise can help to program your subconscious mind for success and keep you concentrated on the positive issues of your sweats.

7. Celebrate the trip: Remember, change is not a destination, it's a continuous trip of growth and self- discovery. Enjoy the process of learning new goods, exploring new habits, and getting to know yourself. Take time to savor the small triumphs and celebrate the overall progress you're making. Erecting a positive mindset for change is not always easy, but it's essential for long-term success.

By incorporating these tips into your routine, you can cultivate a further auspicious outlook, overcome challenges, and ultimately achieve your asked transformation. Remember to believe in yourself, celebrate your progress, and enjoy the trip!

• Overcoming Mental Barriers to Exercise

We all know exercise is good for us. But when it comes to actually lacing up our lurkers, internal hurdles can trip us up hastily than a loose shoelace. Fear, mistrustfulness, and procrastination can turn the routine into a torture chamber, leaving us feeling defeated before we indeed begin. But sweat not, fitness friend!

Here are some ways to outwit your inner critic and overcome those internal walls to exercise.

1. Reframe your thinking: Ditch the" no pain, no gain" intelligence. Exercise should be pleasurable, not excruciating. Choose conditioning you actually like, whether it's dancing, swimming, or brisk walks in nature.
2. Start small and celebrate: Do not overwhelm yourself with hour-long spa sessions. Begin with manageable pretensions, like a 10 minute walk or a simple yoga routine. As you gain confidence, gradually increase the intensity and duration. Remember, every step counts!.
3. Befriend the chum system: Find a drill mate or join a group fitness class. Social support can boost provocation, make exercises further pleasurable, and hold you responsible. Plus, participating triumphs are twice as sweet!.
4. Silence the inner critic: We all have that voice-tail misgivings in our observance. Challenge those negative studies with positive declarations. Remind yourself of your strengths and why you are starting this trip in the first place.
5. Track your progress: Seeing your advancements, no matter how small, is an important motivator. Keep a fitness journal or use a fitness shamus to cover your progress. Witnessing your own growth will fuel your desire to keep going.
6. Embrace the power of music: Produce a drill playlist that pumps you up and gets your bases moving. The right music can take your mind off fatigue and fit a cure of energy into your exercise routine.
7. Make it accessible: Record your exercises in advance and treat them like important movables. Pack your spa bag the night ahead or keep drill clothes readily available at home. Removing obstacles makes it easier to stick to your plans.
8. Listen to your body: Do not push yourself to the point of injury. Overtraining can lead to collapse and unhinge your progress.

Remember, exercise is about feeling good, not looking a certain way. Be patient with yourself, celebrate your successes, and most importantly, have fun! Flash back, the body you have moments is the perfect starting point for an amazing adventure. So lace up your shoes, put on your smile, and conquer that mental barrier and for all!

Chapter 3: A Reason to Change

We all know the drill. The alarm timepiece riots and the lure of the snooze button becomes nearly infectious. But what if there was a way to reignite your fitness trip, not with guilt or obligation, but with the sheer joy of movement? Remember the Feeling? Perhaps it was dancing like nothing was watching, the exhilaration of conquering a grueling hike, or the exhilarating freedom of a bike lift through the wind. Rediscover that joy, and watch your exercises transfigure from a dreaded task to an eagerly anticipated adventure.

1. Unleash Your Inner Explorer : Ditch the spa pattern and explore the endless possibilities of movement. Take a salsa class, climb a gemstone wall, or join a comber derby platoon. Step outside your comfort zone and embrace the exhilaration of learning a new commodity. Your body will thank you for the challenge, and your spirit will soar with a sense of accomplishment.
2. Move to Your Own Groove: Forget the pressure of chasing trends or emulating fitness influencers. Find what makes you move, whether it's a gentle yoga inflow in the morning sun or a 10 minute exercise session in your living room. Listen to your body, admire its measures, and let your own unique energy guide your exercises.
3. Embrace the Journey: Finding your reason to change is not about achieving a specific thing or fitting into a certain earth. It's about falling in love with the process of movement. Celebrate the small victories, savor the feeling of strength and vitality, and connect with the joy of being alive in your body.

So, gutter the guilt, silence the inner critic, and rediscover the magic of movement. Let your trip be guided by the symphony of your breath and the pure joy of feeling your body move.

The path to a fulfilling fitness trip isn't about reaching a destination, but about rediscovering the wonder of the cotillion . Remember, every step, every jump, every beat of your heart is a festivity of life. Move with joy, move with purpose, and move with the unwavering belief that your body is capable of amazing effects. The spark you've been searching for is formerly within you. It's time to unleash it and let your fitness trip be a show of movement, joy, and endless possibilities.

• **Connecting Goals to Long-Term Well-being**

Forget fad diets and quick fixes. True well-being isn't just a sculpted physique or a number on the scale. It's a vibrant tapestry woven from threads of physical, mental, and emotional health. So, how do we ensure our fitness goals become part of this vibrant tapestry, not just fleeting threads that unravel with time?

1. Align Your Focus: Ditch the "beach bod" mentality. Instead, connect your fitness goals to deeper well-being ambitions. Want more energy for adventures? Aim for increased stamina. Craving better sleep? Prioritize stress-busting workouts. Link your movements to the life you long to live.
2. Nourish from Within: Forget crash diets and processed shortcuts. Fuel your body with whole, nutritious foods that nourish not just your muscles, but your brain and spirit too. Healthy eating habits lay the foundation for sustained energy, mental clarity, and overall well-being.
3. Embrace the Power of Meditation: Integrate meditation into your movement. Focus on your breath, connect with your body's sensations, and savor the joy of movement. Mindful exercise reduces stress, enhances focus, and creates a holistic approach to well-being.
4. Make it a Lifestyle, Not a Chore: Forget temporary resolutions. Integrate movement into your daily life. Take the stairs, do mini-workouts throughout the day, find active hobbies. Turn fitness into a natural part of your rhythm, not a forced chore, making well-being a sustainable way of life.

Remember, weaving fitness goals into the tapestry of well-being is an ongoing process. It's not about achieving perfection, but about nurturing a healthy relationship with your body, mind, and spirit. So, listen to your needs, celebrate your victories, and find joy in the movement. When you do, you'll create a vibrant tapestry of well-being that lasts far beyond the next gym session.

Chapter 4: You Are What You Do: Start Right Now

Forget waiting for Monday "motivation" or the "perfect time" to start. Your future fitness isn't a distant dream, it's woven into the fabric of every choice you make, every step you take, right now.

1. Ditch the All-or-Nothing Trap: Start small, with something achievable right now. A brisk walk, a yoga pose in your living room, even five minutes of jumping jacks – every action, however humble, is a thread woven into the tapestry of your future fitness.
2. Move Like You Mean It: Forget autopilot routines. Inject intention into your movement. Feel the ground beneath your feet, the wind against your skin, the power in your muscles. Conscious movement ignites your inner athlete, building momentum for a lifelong journey of well-being.
3. Nourish, Don't Deprive: Forget restrictive diets and calorie counting. Choose foods that energize and nourish your body and soul. A healthy snack right now is an investment in your future strength and clarity. Fuel your body wisely, and it will reward you with sustained energy and confidence.
4. Listen to Your Body: Forget pushing through pain or ignoring fatigue. Be your body's advocate. Take rest days when needed, stretch with intention, and celebrate the quiet strength of recovery. Every conscious choice you make at this moment lays the foundation for a resilient, injury-free future.
5. Surround Yourself with Positivity: Forget toxic comparisons and negativity. Find your peers, online or offline, who cheer you on, share your passion, and inspire you to move. Positive energy is contagious, and the right support system can propel you towards a future brimming with health and happiness.
6. Make it Fun, Not a Chore: Forget about dreading the treadmill or forcing yourself through grueling drills. Find activities you genuinely enjoy, from dancing to swimming to climbing. Movement that sparks joy fuels your desire to move, paving the way for a future where fitness feels like a celebration, not a struggle.
7. Remember, Progress, Not Perfection: Forget the pressure to be perfect. Every stumble, every setback, is a lesson learned, a thread woven into the

tapestry of your growth. Embrace the journey, celebrate the progress, and remember that your future fitness is built, step by step, right now.

You are what you do, one choice, one step, one healthy bite at a time. Your future fitness isn't waiting for some distant start date – it's being woven into every moment, every decision you make right now. So, lace up your shoes, nourish your body, and embrace the joy of movement. The tapestry of your future well-being awaits, vibrant and full of promise, waiting to be crafted with every action you take. Start now, and watch your story unfold.

• The Power of Small, Consistent Actions

Forget overnight metamorphoses and unsustainable actions. True fitness magic lies in the quiet power of small, harmonious conduct, like bitsy vestments weaving a vibrant shade of well- being.

1. Embrace   the   mini-workout: Ditch   the" no   pain,   no   gain" intelligence.Exchange hour-long   spa sessions for bite- sized bursts of movement. Ten minutes of yoga in the morning, a brisk walk during your lunch break, and many bodyweight exercises before bed – each action, still humble, adds a vital thread to your fitness.
2. Make it a Daily Ritual: Forget sporadic bursts of provocation. Integrate movement into your diurnal routine like clockwork. record those mini-workouts, pack your spa bag the night ahead, make healthy choices every mess – thickness is the needle that aches your fitness pretensions into the fabric of your life.
3. Focus on Progress, Not Perfection: Ditch the pressure to be indefectible. Accept that lapses are ineluctable vestments in your shade. Learn from them, acclimate your course, and keep moving. Celebrate progress, no matter how small, for it's the steady drip that fills the well of long- term success.
4. Befriend the Power of Habit: Forget constant restraint battles. Turn healthy choices into automatic vestments in your shade. Take the stairs rather than

the elevator, choose water over sugary drinks, pack nutritional snacks. Little habits, once woven into your routine, come out as the best version of well- being.

5. Find Joy in the Movement: Explore conditioning you authentically enjoy, from dancing to swimming to gemstone climbing. Movement that sparks joy energies your desire to move, weaving vestments of happiness and provocation into your fitness trip.

6. Connect with Your Body: Be present in your movement. Feel the ground beneath your bases, the wind against your skin, the strength in your muscles. This aware connection weaves vestments of mindfulness and appreciation into your shade, making fitness a trip of self- discovery.

7. Celebrate the Ripple Effect: Forget insulated conduct. Every small step you take sends ripples of well- being. The energy you gain, the choices you inspire, the positivity you radiate – these are vestments woven into the larger shade of your community, your family, your world. Start small, be harmonious, and celebrate the trip. These are the vestments that weave the vibrant shade of fitness, not a transitory trend, but a sustainable, joyous way of life.

Every bite- sized drill, every healthy choice, every step you take is an investment in your future well- being. So, embrace the power of small, harmonious conduct, and watch your fitness story unfold, thread by thread, into a vibrant shade of health, happiness, and well- being.

Chapter 5: Starting Points and Goals for the Less Active, Obese, and Elderly

Forget one- size- fits- all routines and torture at the gym. Fitness is not just for spa rats and marathon runners. It's a vibrant shade woven by people of all shapes, sizes, and periods. Then is how to find your own starting point and set attainable pretensions, no matter where you're on your trip

For the Less Active:

1. Start small, celebrate big: Ditch the pressure of hour-long exercises. Begin with 10 minute walks, gentle stretches, or president exercises. Every step counts! Find the fun.
2. Forget boring routines: Explore moments you enjoy, like dancing, swimming, or gardening. Movement should not feel like a chore.
3. Pay attention to your body: Know your limitations. Take rest days when demanded and prioritize gentle movement over pushing yourself too hard.
4. Set SMART decisions : Make your decisions Specific, Measurable, Attainable, Applicable, and Time- bound. Aim for short, attainable mileposts, like walking for 30 twinkles three times a week.

For the obese:

1. Focus on health, not weight:Focusing on health rather than weight promotes a holistic approach to well-being. Prioritizing nutritious food, regular exercise, and mental wellness contributes to overall health, irrespective of body size or shape. It's about embracing habits that nourish both the body and mind.
2. Find your support system: Surround yourself with positive and encouraging people who celebrate your progress. Find a drill class or join a fitness class for support and provocation.
3. Set achievable goals:Track advancements in how you feel, not just what you weigh. Aim for climbing stairs with lower trouble, walking pain-free for longer distances, or feeling further confident in your body. Track small triumphs like climbing stairs with lower trouble, walking longer distances,

or feeling further confident in your body. These mileposts fuel your provocation.

For the Elderly:

1. Stay active, stay independent: Maintain mobility and strength for everyday tasks. Simple exercises like president syllables, balance exercises, and light walks can make a big difference.
2. Make it social: Join a elderly fitness class, take group walks in the demesne, or find conditioning you can enjoy with musketeers and family. Social commerce boosts provocation and well- being.
3. Consult your doctor: Listen to your doctor before starting any new exercise program. They can help you conform your routine to your specific requirements and limitations.

Remember, fitness is a trip, not a destination. Start where you are, celebrate every step, and concentrate on progress, not perfection. Your body is capable of amazing effects, no matter your age or current fitness position. Embrace the joy of movement, and watch your own vibrant shade of health and well- being unfold, one step at a time.

• Assessing Your Current Activity Level

Forget Labels like" unfit" or" unattractive" Every trip begins with a step, and understanding your current movement habits is the first step towards a healthier, happier you. also is how to assess your exertion position, whether you're just starting out, managing weight, or navigating life's after chapters.

For the Less Active:

1. Beyond the gym tasks count!:Track how important you walk, climb stairs, or do chores like gardening. Every bit of movement contributes to your overall exertion position. hear to your breath Pay attention to how you feel during everyday exertion. Can you talk comfortably while walking? Do you get

winded climbing stairs? These suggestions can help gauge your current fitness.

2. Be true to yourself: Start by admitting your current routine, without judgment. This honest assessment is your heliport for making positive changes.

For the obese:

1. Focus on gentle movements: Ditch the pressure of violent exercises. Start with small, manageable activities you enjoy, like short walks, light stretches, or chairman exercises. Listen to your body and avoid anything that causes pain or discomfort.

2. Track your way: Invest in a pedometer or use a fitness app to cover your quotidian way. Aim for gradual increases week by week, celebrating milestones along the way.

3. Consult your doctor: Before starting any new exercise program, go through your decisions and limitations with your doctor. They can give substantiated guidance and ensure your safety.

For the Elderly:

1. Embrace movement: Focus on incorporating exertion into your routine. Take the stairs rather than the elevator, or do simple exercises while watching TV. Every bit counts! Listen to your body. Pay attention to your energy situations and adjust your exertion accordingly. Take rest days when demanded and prioritize balance and harshness exercises to maintain mobility.

2. Find joy in movement: Choose movements you genuinely enjoy, like dancing to music, swimming in a pool, or taking gentle walks in nature.Movement should be an enriching experience, not a chore. Assessing your exertion position is not about judging or labeling yourself. It's about gaining a clear understanding of your starting point so you can set attainable goals and embark on a sustainable trip towards a healthier, happier you. Celebrate every step, every bit of movement, and watch your own vibrant shade of well- being unfold, one movement at a time.

• Fun Smart Nutrition Ideas

Forget Mellow diets and restrictive rules. Nourishing your body for movement should be a succulent adventure, not a chore.

Here are some fun and smart nutrition ideas for the less active, fat, and elderly to fuel their unique expeditions.

For the Less Active:

1. Snack smart: Ditch empty calories. conclude for bite- sized bursts of energy like colorful fruit skewers, hummus and veggie ladles, or homemade trail mix with nuts and seeds.
2. Spice up your water: Plain water can get boring. Invest it with fruits, gravies, or cucumber for a stimulating twist.
3. Ditch the TV bowl: Set the table, light candles, and play upbeat music. Turn mealtime into a fun social event, indeed if it's just for one!

For the obese :

1. Prioritize protein: It keeps you feeling full and helps make muscle. Include protein in every mess, like eggs for breakfast, grilled funk for lunch, and lentil haze for dinner.
2. Rainbow on your plate: Fill your plate with colorful fruits and vegetables. They're low in calories and packed with nutrients your body needs. Aim for a different color every day!
3. Exchange sweet for savory: Ditch sticky treats. Indulge in naturally sweet fruits like berries and melons, or try baked apples with cinnamon for a warm, comforting delicacy .

For the Elderly:

1. Focus on fiber: It keeps you feeling full and regular. conclude for whole grains like brown rice and quinoa, tire and lentils, and cornucopia of fruits and vegetables.
2. Hydrate, hydrate, hydrate: Dehydration can be sneaky in aged grown- ups. Carry a portable water bottle and belt throughout the day. Add a squeeze of

lemon for a stimulating twist. Try mini sandwiches, yogurt parfaits, or veggie sticks with hummus for accessible, nutritive snacks. There is no any-size- fits- all approach to food. Have fun, and discover what makes you feel good. Food should be a source of joy, not stress.

Celebrate every healthy choice, big or small, and watch your body thrive on the succulent energy you give. Your path to well- being begins with you, so make it a beautiful adventure!

Chapter 6: Detailed Diets and Exercising Plan

• Creating Balanced and Sustainable Diets

Ditch the style diets and calorie counting! Creating a balanced and sustainable diet is not about privation, it's about smart choices that nourish your body and soul, right now and for the long haul. Then is how to create a balanced and sustainable diet.

1. Go Rainbow, Not Restrictive: Fill your plate with vibrant fruits and vegetables of all colors – each tinge packing unique nutrients for a healthy symphony of well- being.

2. Befriend the Whole Grains: Ditch carbs. Exchange white chuck and pasta for whole- wheat options, brown rice, quinoa, and oats. They'll keep you fuller for longer, fueling your energy situations all day.

3. Make Protein Your Partner: Include protein in every bite, from eggs for breakfast to lentils for lunch to grilled funk for regale. It builds muscle, keeps you feeling satisfied, and supports a healthy metabolism.

4. Do not sweat the Fat: Ditch the fat-free mode. Choose healthy fats like avocado, nuts, seeds, and olive oil painting. They keep your brain sharp, your heart happy.

5. Hydrate, Hydrate, Hydrate: Forget sticky drinks. Make water your stylish friend. inoculate it with fruits, sauces, or cucumber for a stimulating twist. perk points for a fancy ice cell charger with frozen berries!

6. Take your time when eating: Ditch the autopilot eating. Savor your food, chew sluggishly, and connect with the flavors and textures. Taking your time when eating helps you appreciate your aliment and avoid gluttony.

7. Cook More, Dine Less: Ditch the takeout habit. Make simple, healthy meals at home. It's cheaper, healthier, and gives you control over your constituents. Plus, cuisine can be a fun exercise! .

8. Listen to Your Body: Ditch the rigid schedules. Eat when you are empty, stop when you are full. Trust your body's natural signals and do not force yourself to eat when you are not feeling it.

9. Make it Delicious, Not Depriving: Ditch the mellow options. Explore spices, sauces, and cooking ways to make healthy food scrumptious and instigative. Your taste kids will thank you!

Remember, progress not perfection. Ditch the guilt passages. Small, harmonious choices add up. Celebrate every healthy plate, every shifted soda pop for water, every step towards a more balanced, sustainable you. erecting a balanced and sustainable diet is a trip, not a destination. Embrace the joy of healthy eating, hear to your body, and watch your vibrant shade of well- being unfold, suck by succulent bites.

• **Tailoring Exercise Plans to Individual Needs**

Your fitness journey deserves a bespoke tapestry, woven with threads of activity that suit your unique needs and desires. Here's how to tailor your exercise plan for a vibrant, personalized well-being:

1. Do not listen to Trends: Forget chasing fads or comparing yourself to others. Tune into your body's whispers. Enjoy high-intensity workouts? Embrace them! Prefer gentle yoga flows? Do it! Prioritize movement that sparks joy and fuels your passion.

2.Befriend Your Fitness Level: Forget pushing yourself to exhaustion. Start where you are, with activities you can comfortably manage. Walking, swimming, dancing – every thread, however humble, strengthens your fitness tapestry.

3.Make it Mini, Make it Daily: Integrate movement into your routine like clockwork. Schedule mini-workouts, pack your gym bag the night before, choose healthy snacks – consistency weaves your goals into the very fabric of your life.

4.Embrace Variety, Spice Up Your Routine: Forget monotonous drills. Keep your body and mind engaged with diverse activities. Mix cardio with strength training, try a new yoga pose, explore interval training – variety keeps your workouts fresh and exciting.

5.Be Flexible, Listen to Your Limits: Forget pushing through pain or ignoring fatigue. Respect your limitations. Take rest days when needed, adjust your intensity, and prioritize mindful movement that nourishes your body.

Remember, your fitness plan is a living tapestry, constantly evolving and adapting to your needs. Listen to your body, celebrate your victories, and find joy in the movement. Every step you take, every choice you make, is a thread woven into the vibrant tapestry of your well-being. So, embrace the possibilities, personalize your workout, and watch your unique fitness story unfold, one movement at a time.

Chapter 7: Add Practical Ways to Help You Stay Fit

• Incorporating Exercise into Daily Routines

Weaving movement into your daily tapestry does not need to be a dramatic overhaul. Then is how to seamlessly blend fitness into your everyday life

1. Make Mini Mighty: Ditch the pressure of hour-long exercises. Embrace bite-sized bursts of movement. Ten twinkles of yoga before bed, a brisk walk during your lunch break, though small, strengthens your fitness fabric.

2. Befriend the Stairs: Ditch the elevator. Embrace the challenge of stairs. Take them two at a time, hop every other step. Turning everyday tasks into mini-workouts adds up, one stair at a time.

3. Transfigure Chores into Cardio: Ditch the autopilot cleaning. Turn housework into a cotillion party. Blast music while vacuuming, mop like you are gliding on ice, dust with jabs – every clean reach becomes a calorie- burning burst.

4. Embrace Active Errands: Ditch the auto for short passages. Walk, bike, or rollerblade to the grocery store, coffee shop, or library. Turn errands intomini-adventures, exploring your neighborhood on bottom and feeling the wind in your hair.

5. Befriend the Commercial Break: Ditch the settee potato routine. Use television breaks for quick bursts of movement. Do jumping jacks, syllables, or push- ups during commercials, making your screen time a sneaky fitness session.

6. Make Meetings Mobile: Ditch the static conference apartments. Hold walking meetings, take breaks for group stretches, or suggest active brainstorming sessions. Get your ideas flowing .

7. Park Farther Down: Ditch the front- door honor. Park further down and enjoy the redundant way. Turn parking into amini-hike, adding distance and sneaky movement to your daily routine.

Weaving fitness into your daily routine is about small, harmonious choices. Start with one thread, also another, and watch your shade of well- being bloom, vibrant and alive. Every step, every active choice, is a masterpiece in the timber. So, embrace the possibilities, move with intention, and watch your everyday routine transfigure into a playground for your well- being.

• Finding Enjoyable Activities for Long-Term Commitment

Forget chasing fleeting trends or forcing yourself through dreaded routines. Lasting joy in movement lies in weaving threads of activities you genuinely love into the tapestry of your life. Here's how to find activities that ignite your passion and keep you moving, year after year:

1. Tap into Your Inner Child: Ditch the "grown-up" pressure. Remember the activities that set your heart racing as a kid? Climbing trees, dancing uninhibited, swimming like a mermaid – rediscover the pure joy of movement without limitations.

2. Explore the Great Outdoors: Ditch the gym walls. Embrace the vast playground of nature. Hike through sun-dappled forests, paddle across shimmering lakes, cycle through winding trails – nature's beauty fuels your spirit and strengthens your body.

3. Listen to Your Body's Symphony: Ditch the one-size-fits-all mentality. Tune into your body's whispers. Crave the rhythm of dance? Salsa your heart out! Yearn for the quiet focus of yoga? Unfurl your mat and flow. Movement that resonates with your being sparks long-term commitment.

4.Embrace the Spirit of Play: Ditch the seriousness. Turn fitness into a playground for your inner child. Play hopscotch, jump rope like you're ten again, have snowball fights in winter – rediscover the simple joy of playful movement, and your body will thank you.

5.Dance to Your Own Beat: Ditch the pressure to conform. Celebrate your unique rhythm. Love heavy metal drumming? Rock out with a drumstick and air guitar!

Find joy in movement that expresses your individuality, not someone else's definition of fitness.

6.Fuel Your Curiosity: Ditch the boredom of repetitive routines. Explore new activities every season. Try kayaking in summer, rock climbing in fall, ice skating in winter – keep your body and mind engaged with fresh challenges and discoveries.

7.Make it a Multisensory Feast: Engage all your senses in your movement. Feel the wind against your skin on a bike ride, smell the pine needles on a hike, hear the music pulse through your body in a dance class – sensory experiences weave richness into your fitness journey.

So, embrace the possibilities, explore with curiosity, and watch your tapestry of movement unfold, vibrant and ever-evolving, fueled by the joy of activities you truly love. Remember, lasting commitment isn't about forcing yourself, it's about finding activities that make your soul sing – and keep you moving, year after year.

● Fun Workout Ideas

Forget the treadmill treadmill. Ditch the repetitive routines! Your workout shouldn't feel like homework, it should be a playground for your inner child (and grown-up self, of course). Here are some fun ideas to shake up your sweat session and paint your fitness journey with vibrant colors:

1. Dance Party Blitz: Blast your favorite tunes and let loose! Channel your inner rockstar, Bollywood dancer, or salsa king/queen. No choreography required, just let the music move you. Bonus points for themed dance parties: 80s aerobics anyone?

2. Parkour Playground: Turn your city jungle into an obstacle course. Climb stairs, hop curbs, vault benches – unleash your inner parkour artist and navigate the urban landscape with playful agility. Just remember, safety first!

3. Flash Mob Fitness: Surprise your friends and family with a spontaneous workout session. Bust out some squats in the park, hold a plank in the living room, or do

jumping jacks on the sidewalk. Spread the fitness cheer and inspire others to join the fun!

4. Nature Quest: Lace up your shoes and explore the green side of town. Hike, bike, or jog through nature trails, chasing butterflies and soaking in the fresh air. Turn it into a scavenger hunt, collecting leaves, acorns, or colorful pebbles along the way.

5. Board Game Bonanza: Who says games can't be sweaty? Dust off your old favorites and add a fitness twist. Do jumping jacks for every wrong answer in Monopoly, hold planks during Scrabble turns, or race around the board in Twister. Laughter and movement guaranteed!

6. Aquatic Adventures: Dive into the cool embrace of water. Swimming, kayaking, or paddleboarding are refreshing workouts that engage your whole body. Bonus points for synchronized swimming routines with friends – mermaids, anyone?

7. Animal Kingdom Workout: Unleash your inner animal with animal-inspired movements. Bear crawls, frog jumps, bird dogs – mimic the motions and feel the power surge through your muscles. Roar like a lion after each set for extra motivation!

8. Kitchen Olympics: Turn your kitchen into a fitness arena. Carry watermelons like weights, do lunges while mixing batter, or hold wall sits while waiting for the oven. Multitasking at its finest (and tastiest)!

9. Music Video Mashup: Recreate your favorite music videos, from Beyonce's "Crazy in Love" to Michael Jackson's "Thriller." Learn the moves, crank up the volume, and let your inner performer shine. Bonus points for costumes and props!

10. Flashback Fun: Dust off the oldies! Play hopscotch, jump rope, or hula hoop like you did as a kid. Rediscover the simple joys of movement and relive the carefree laughter of childhood.

Remember, fitness should be fun, not a chore. Embrace the silliness, explore the possibilities, and watch your workout sessions transform into vibrant tapestries of laughter, movement, and well-being. So, unleash your inner child, get creative, and let the fun fitness games begin!

Chapter 8: Action Points to Remember

• Recap of Key Concepts

1. Start small, dream big: Embrace small actions, celebrate progress, and watch your fitness goals unfold.
2. Befriend the power of habit: Ditch willpower battles, turn healthy choices into automatic threads in your tapestry.
3. Find joy in the movement: Explore activities you love, from dancing to swimming, and fuel your desire to move.
4. Listen to your body: Respect your limitations, adapt your routine, and prioritize mindful movement.
5. Celebrate non-scale victories: Focus on increased energy, better sleep, and confidence gains, not just numbers.
6. Tailor your goals, personalize your plan: Craft goals that fit your needs, choose activities you enjoy, and make fitness your own adventure.
7. Fuel your body, nourish your soul: Prioritize whole foods, colorful fruits and vegetables, and make mealtime a mindful joy.
8. Variety is the spice of life: Mix up your workouts, explore new activities, and keep your body and mind engaged.
9. Find your tribe, move together: Connect with like-minded individuals, share the joy of movement, and support each other's journeys.
10. Remember, progress, not perfection: Celebrate every step, every healthy choice, and embrace the ever-evolving tapestry of your well-being.

Let these threads guide you, inspire you, and empower you to weave your own vibrant story of health, happiness, and joyful movement. Remember, the journey begins with a single step, and every choice you make, every thread you add, strengthens the magnificent tapestry of your well-being.

- **Setting Weekly and Monthly Milestones**

Weekly Wonders: Fun & Feasible Fitness Goals

Monday Motivation:

1. Sunrise Stretch: Hail the day with a 10- minute yoga flux outside. Feel the sun on your skin and gobble some fresh air.
2. Walk & Talk: Exchange phone calls for walking meetings with associates. Get your way in while catching up – double win!
3. Staircase Sprint: Ditch the elevator, conquer the stairs twice a day. Make it a quick challenge, or add some playful jumping jacks at the top for spare oomph.

Tuesday Twists:

1. Strength Seeker: Hit the gym or home for a 20- minute strength training session.
2. Target different muscle groups each day, feel your power grow!
3. Dance Delight: Blast your favorite warbles and let loose! Dance it out for 15 beats, demonstrative and joyful.
4. Posture Power: Focus on aligning your spine, stretching your shoulders, and holding your head high throughout the day. Feel the confidence boost!

Wednesday Wellness:

1. Hydration Hero: Challenge yourself to drink 10 specs of water moment. invest it with fruits, gravies, or cucumber for a stimulating twist. Stay doused, conquer the day!
2. Apprehensive Munching: Pack a healthy lunch rather of grabbing takeout. Include colorful fruits and vegetables, whole grains, and spare protein. Nourish your body, stay energized!
3. Tech Time- Out: Take a screen break after every hour. Do some eye stretches, walk around the block, or simply close your eyes and breathe. Give your mind and body amini- detox!

Thursday charges:

1. Team Up: Call a friend or family member for a drill session. Join a fitness class, play active games in the demesne, or challenge each other to plank holds.
2. Kitchen Cardio: Transfigure drawing into a calorie- burning burst! dance while vacuuming, do lunges while mopping, or thickset while putting away dishes. Multitasking at its finest!
3. Skillful way: Exercise a new movement skill this week. Master a balance disguise in yoga, learn a jump rope trick, or perfect a tennis serve. Small strides, big progress!

Friday Fiesta:

1. Fit & Fun Friday: End the week with a fun exertion that gets your heart pumping. Go for a rollerblading adventure, try rock climbing with buddies, or join a community dance class. Celebrate movement, feel the joy!
2. Rest & Reflect: Take a comforting bath, read a good book, or enjoy a quiet evening with loved ones. Recharge your batteries, come back strong coming week!

Bonus: Track your progress throughout the week. Celebrate every corner, no matter how small. Award yourself for achieving your pretensions, keep the provocation flowing!

Monthly Marvels: Mastering Milestones Step-by-Step

1. Challenge Champion: Choose a physical exertion challenge for the month, like running an athlete, doing 100 push- ups daily, or completing a yoga disguise challenge. Set yourself small, attainable diurnal targets and track your progress. Celebrate each accomplishment, and conquer the overall challenge at the end of the month!
2. Skill spotlight: Pick a new fitness skill you'd like to master this month. Focus on perfecting your form in a specific exercise, learning a new dance

routine, or learning a yoga sequence. devote specific practice time each week, track your progress, and validate your chops blossom!

3. Healthy Habits Hero: Choose a healthy habit you want to solidify this month, like drinking enough water, mess preparing for the week, or getting to bed ahead. Set diurnal monuments, track your progress, and reward yourself for consistency. Make it a fun challenge, and let healthy choices become part of your life!

4. Community Connection: Join a fitness club, online community, or team over with a drill buddy this month. Partake your pretensions, offer support, and hold each other responsible. Social commerce and goad make fitness a more enjoyable and satisfying trip. So, there you have it – a vibrant toolkit for weaving the shade of your well- being, thread by thread, week by week, month by month.

Remember , there's no one - size- fits- all path to fitness. Embrace the joy of movement, explore your heartstrings, and set pretensions that inspire, not blackjack. Celebrate small triumphs, track your progress, and reward yourself for consistency. Above all, have fun! Let your diurnal cautions and monthly sensations be stepping monuments, not stumbling blocks. adapt them to your unique conditions, hear to your body, and find activities that sets your soul on fire. With each movement, with each healthy choice, you strengthen the vestments of your well- being, creating a masterpiece of health, happiness, and vibrant life.

Go forth, explore, move, and celebrate! The shade of your well- being awaits, staying to be woven with the vibrant vestments of your own joyful trip

da

CONCLUSION

Dear beginner, your fitness journey isn't a sprint, it's a vibrant tapestry woven with threads of small, sustainable choices. Celebrate the non-scale victories: the extra pep in your step, the deeper sleep, the confidence that blossoms as you conquer stairs with ease. Every movement, every healthy bite, is a thread strengthening the magnificent tapestry of your well-being.

Remember, progress, not perfection, is your mantra. Listen to your body, listen to your soul. Find activities that spark joy, not dread. Dance like nobody's watching, walk instead of driving, embrace the playful spirit of a child. Let's face it, who said burpees have to be fun?

This guide is your compass, not your cage. Adapt it, bend it, make it your own. Set goals that whisper "challenge" but never scream "torture." Find your tribe, move together, laugh together, sweat together. And most importantly, celebrate every milestone, big or small. A pat on the back, a relaxing bath, a good book – reward yourself for weaving your healthy habits into the fabric of your life.

This journey isn't about reaching some distant finish line. It's about the joy of movement, the power of mindful choices, the confidence that blooms with each healthy step. So, take a deep breath, beginner, and step onto your path. The tapestry of your well-being awaits, ready to be woven with the vibrant threads of your own joyful, sustainable, and yes, absolutely achievable fitness goals.

Go forth, move, and celebrate! You've got this.

REVIEW PAGE

Dear Reviewer,

I hope this message finds you well. I am reaching out to request your valuable feedback on Callie's latest work, Achieving realistic fitness goals: A guide to Sustainable fitness goals for beginners. As a respected reviewer in the fitness field, your insights would greatly contribute to the understanding and appreciation of Callie's unique perspective on Achieving realistic fitness goals: A guide to Sustainable fitness goals for beginners.

Callie is a fitness expert with a focus on sustainable fitness goals, and her recent publication delves into innovative approaches to achieving long-term health and wellness. The comprehensive nature of her work is intended to resonate with a diverse audience, and your discerning review could provide potential readers with valuable insights.

If you are interested and available, we would be happy to provide you with a complimentary copy of Achieving realistic fitness goals: A guide to Sustainable fitness goals for beginners.

for your review. Your expertise and thoughtful evaluation would be immensely beneficial in bringing attention to the important ideas presented in this work.

Please let us know if you are willing to undertake this review, and we will promptly arrange for a copy to be sent to you. Thank you for considering our request, and we look forward to the possibility of your involvement.

Best regards,

Callie M. Henley.